Dear Parents,

Raising a family is not an easy task. Sometimes we are so busy taking care of others that we forget to take care of ourselves. It is important to take some time to unwind and re-energize ourselves. Whether you are a stay at home mom or a working parent, you need to work on having a good mental health to be able to do all your responsibilities and not be overwhelmed.

In this book I will write about what mental health is, why it is important to work on maintaining it, and the steps you can take to work on your specific goal. As a bonus I am including 2 plans that have worked for me. These plans are now part of my routine.

Hope you find this guide helpful!

Ana Soto

Table of Contents

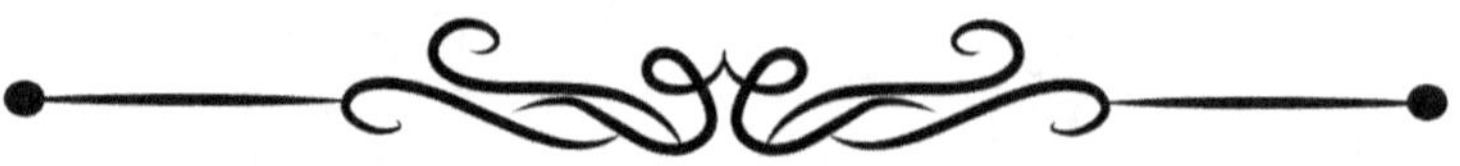

Chapter 1
Mental Health

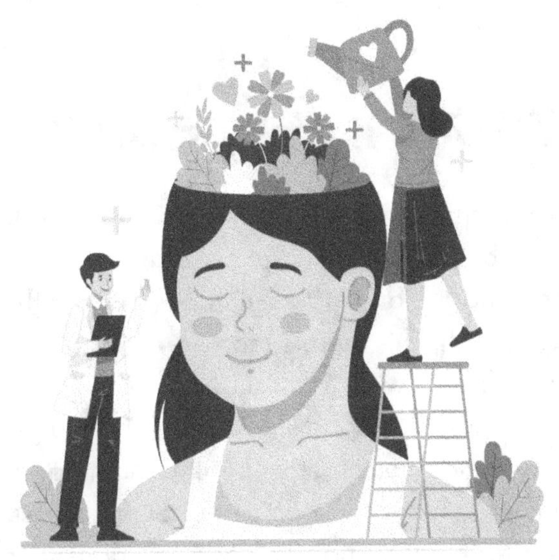

What is mental health?

According to the Center of Disease Control and Prevention (CDC), mental health includes the person's emotional, psychological, and social well-being. It influences how we think, how we feel, and how we act to manage stress, others, and make choices. Having good mental health is important for every stage of our lives, from childhood to adulthood.

Why is it important?

Mental health is important for our overall health. We need to be able to manage our state of mind, our stress, and our daily tasks in conjunction with our physical health. This means that we need to take care of our bodies as well. Mental and Physical health go hand in hand. It is important to know that our mental health can guide our physical health and it can change over time. Many factors can affect our health such as family history, eating habits, sleeping habits, our work life, and any economic hardships.

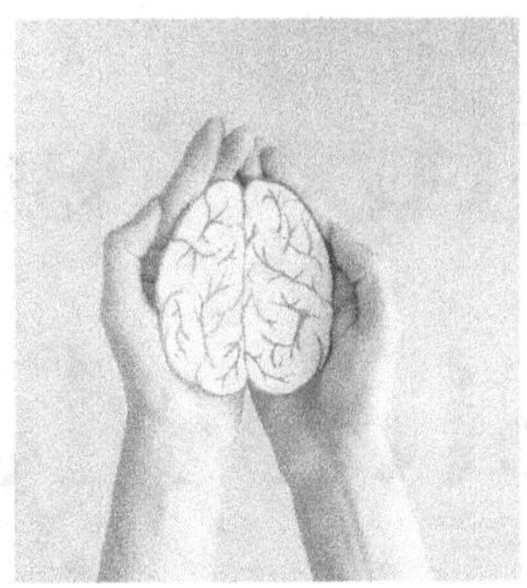

Mental health is considered a taboo topic in many cultures. But, as more information and resources come out, its importance is becoming evident. As parents we really need to be in the right state of mind to be able to do all our responsibilities and stay sane!

In this book I will cover how I have been able to manage my mental health and how you can too! I will discuss strategies that can help you. I will show you five steps that will guide you into having a more positive outlook while you manage your family, your work life, your social life, and your mental health. As parents we wear many hats: moms, dads, friends, nurses, chef, counselors, teachers, and many more!

Chapter 2
Steps for Positive Mental Health

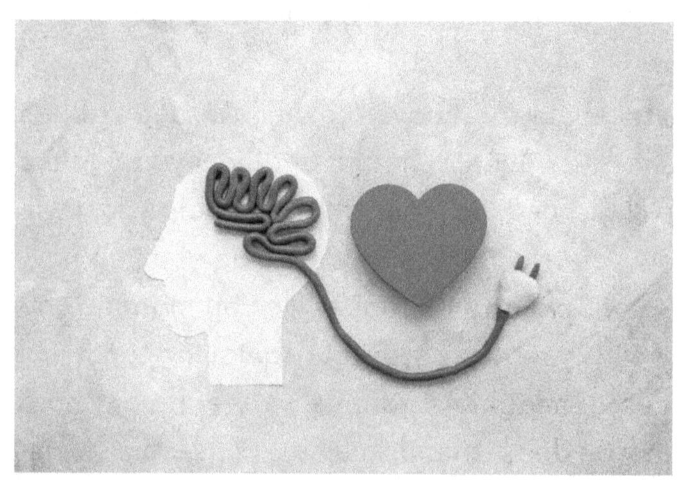

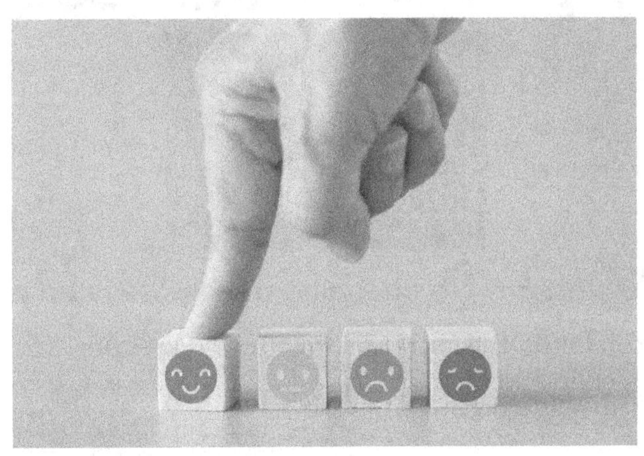

5 steps to work towards your positive mental health goal.

1.	Your SMART Goal
2.	Reflect to motivate
3.	Make a plan
4.	Implement your plan
5.	Reflect to Adjust

Step 1: Your SMART Goal

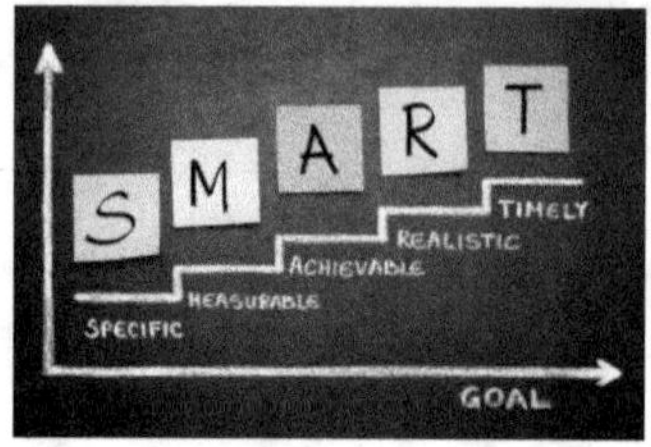

To start any life changing action, we need a goal and thus the why for this goal. We need to know the why behind our decision. This step can be challenging since most of the time we are not specific enough.

Think about the following questions to help you make a SMART (Specific Measurable, Attainable, Relevant, Time-bound) goal. Stating that you want to have good mental health is a start, but this is broad. Your mental health is important, but it takes many forms.

These questions can help you narrow your goal down. It is better to break down a bigger goal into a smaller more specific one. Having a broad goal can be overwhelming but, having a more targeted goal can help you focus and have a better chance at succeeding.

Step 1: Your SMART Goal Continued..

1. What do I want to accomplish?
   - Ex: Reduce stress, cope with anger management, learn how to let go (knowing that some things are out of our control), self - care, boosting your mood, etc.

2. Why do I want to accomplish this? Why is it important?

   Think about the reason you have decided to start: to increase your energy level, your productivity, be healthier, have more self-care, set a good example for your kids, etc.

3. What happens if I do not this?

   Think about what can happen if you do not start taking care of yourself.

4. What is the alternative? Is there any?

   think of how you are right now. Are you happy? Are you free of stress? Do you want to continue being in a state of worry or feeling rushed?

Step 1: Your SMART Goal Continued..

5. How will I know I am succeeding in my goal?
Think about how you know that the methods you
are implementing are working. Are you feeling
less stressed? Are you taking more time for
yourself? Are your reactions to your kid's calmer?
Did you see any difference? etc.

6. How much time am I giving myself to revise and
reflect on my progress?
- When should you reflect? Should I come back
to this plan in a month? 2 months?
Sometimes we need to come back to our
plans and revise. Time is forever changing
but you should always have an end goal.

7. Who can be my support system?
- Think of family and/or friends that can help
you stay on track.

If you have thought about these questions and
have answered them fully and truthfully, then you are
ready for step 2. Again, remember that your mental
health is important. It is okay to take time for
yourself. We, as parents, often forget to do that.

Step 2: Reflect to Motivate.

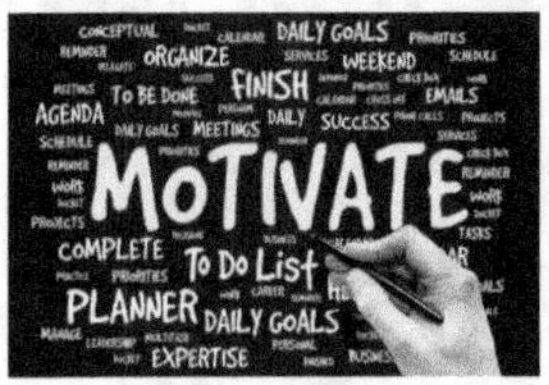

Now that you have your SMART goal, you need to make sure you keep your motivation going. To do this, think about what makes you happy. Close your eyes and really think about what makes you feel relaxed, without worries, without stress, no depression, your energy level was high, and you felt you were in a good place. This can be a specific situation or a time in your life.

Taking the time to really think and reflect is the key to making sure you will stay motivated and be able to create a plan. One strategy is to jot the answer to these questions down or record your answer on your smart device.

Were you....
1. on vacation?
2. reading a book?
3. going out with friends?
4. spending time with family?
5. meditating?
6. able to have time for yourself?

Step 2: Reflect to Motivate Continued.

Now think of what is stopping you from feeling this sense of peace and relaxation.

Do you have:
1. financial problems?
2. specific health problem?
3. life altering event?
4. other people that bring you down?
5. less energy? eating less? eating more?
6. feeling that you never have enough time? Always rushed?
7. Less sleep?

Identifying the time that you felt happy and identifying what is stopping you from feeling this sense of happiness will help you think about your plan. These answers will be the driving force on WHAT you will do and HOW you will do it. These answers will guide your steps. Now you are ready for step 3.

Always remember, your mental health is important. It is okay to take time to better yourself!

Step 3: Make a plan

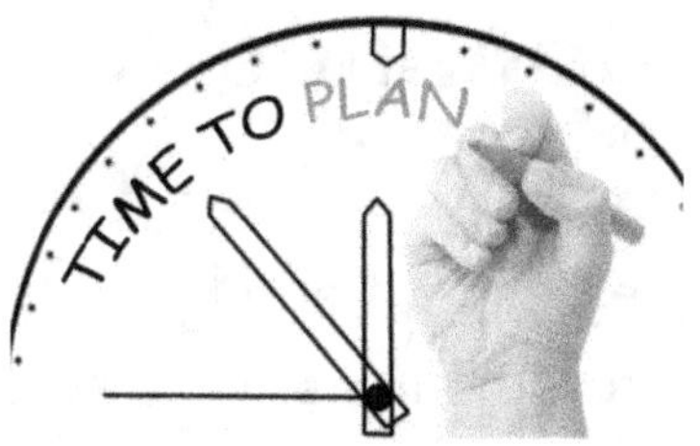

Now that you have identified your goal, have self-reflected on the times that you have felt good with yourself, and the changes that have happened currently in your life, it is time to think on what you will do to better help yourself. What strategies can you implement and when can you implement them? As parents, we are always busy. But like my mother says, "sometimes you need to steal time from yourself for yourself." I know it is easier said than done but, it is possible! You CAN do it!

To make your plan always think of your end goal. You will work backwards to move forward. (sample plans given)

Step 3: Make a plan Continued.

1. Write your goal.
2. Identify strategies that can help you achieve your goal (different strategies discussed in the strategies section)
3. Identify the times in the day or the week when you can implement these strategies (I know you are busy but think of this- you can implement it for 10 minutes once a week- even in the bathroom- It is OK to take time for yourself!)
4. Identify how you will keep track of what you are doing and/or your progress.
5. Identify when you will self-reflect (remember that your goal should be time-bound: 1 month, 2 months, etc.)
6. Identify your support system. (think of that person you can confide in and talk about it)
7. Revise/Adjust your goal or plan to keep going.

After you have made your plan, it is time to execute your plan.

Step 4: Implement your plan.

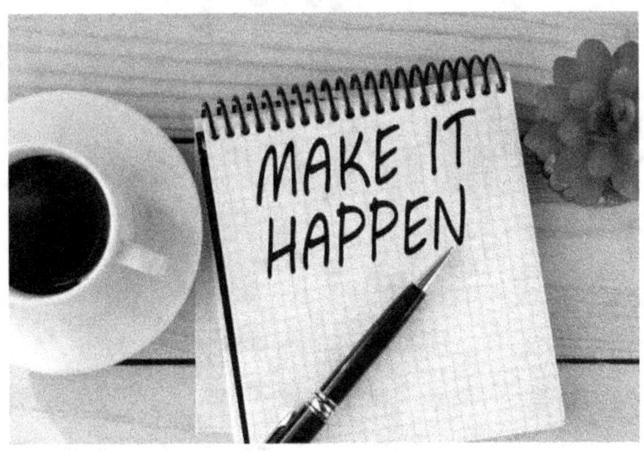

You CAN do this! You deserve to have some time for yourself.

You identified strategies you can do and when it is possible for you to do them. Now all you must do is start. It may feel scary or nervous, and that is okay. Your feelings are valid and are completely normal. Remember that everyone deserves to have a life with minimal stress (I am not going to say no stress since as parents we will always worry and have some stress with our kids. AND this is normal as well!) including you.

Step 5: Reflect to Adjust.

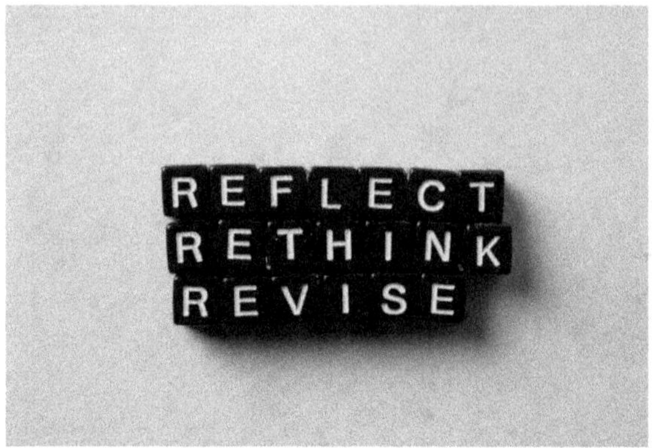

This is the step that most people forget but it is especially important. You need time to reflect and see what has worked and what has not. In this step you will think back to what has occurred during the time when you started till the present.

During this time, you will be able to adjust or tweak your plan OR if it is working, keep at it. If your plan works then eventually it will become a routine, a habit. Good habits are great to have.

Chapter 3
Sample Goals

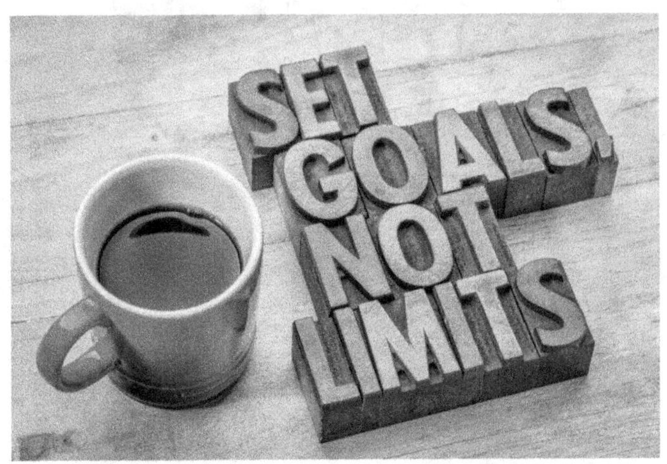

Sample Goal #1
Reducing Stress

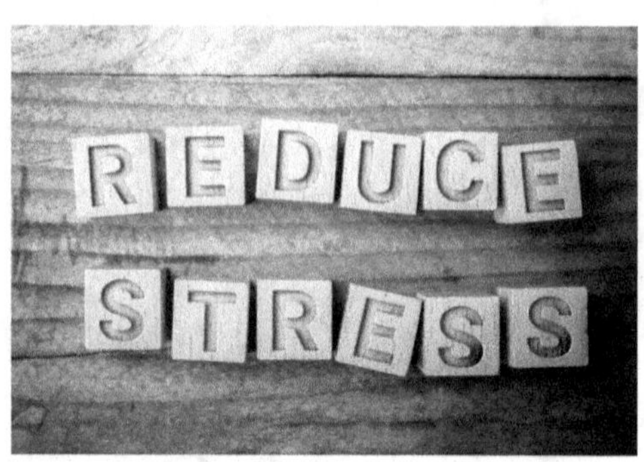

Strategies that can help:

1) Meditation
   a. This can be done daily – several times a day! Practice deep breathing- close your eyes, take a deep breath, hold it in for 10s, then slowly exhale.

2) Get enough sleep.
   a. Our bodies work in healing itself while we sleep. Our brain's nerve cells rewire, allowing us to be able to learn and retain more information. We conserve energy, our cells repair, hormones are released and balanced, and it allows us to think more clearly when we are faced with different situations.

Sample Goal #1 Reducing stress continued...

Strategies that can help:

3) Eat healthily.

Eating a balanced healthy meal can increase your energy and improve your mood thus affecting our brains and other organs in our bodies.

4) Exercise

Walking, swimming, running, or going to the gym will have a positive effect on your body and mind.

5) Read a book.

Choose a topic of interest. buy a book and read several pages a day or a week. Have the right setting. Choose a seat at your house, have a glass of water or wine (up to you!) and just immerse yourself in those pages. Even if you only read five pages, you have worked to have your body and mind in a state of relaxation.

6) Listen to music.

listen to your favorite songs or genre or just a calming sound. While cleaning, cooking, taking shower, going to work, or getting home, it has been said that music is a great stress reliever.

Sample Goal #1 Reducing stress continued...

Strategies that can help:

7) Go out with your friends.
   Can be once a month for an hour or two!
8) Manage your time.
   If you feel always rushed or that you forget to do different things and this increases your stress, then you need time management.
   Create your weekly schedule. Get a dry erase calendar and place it on the fridge. Keep all your appointments in one place (I do this!)
   Have a planner where you can have a daily schedule by the hour.

Sample Goal #2
Self Care

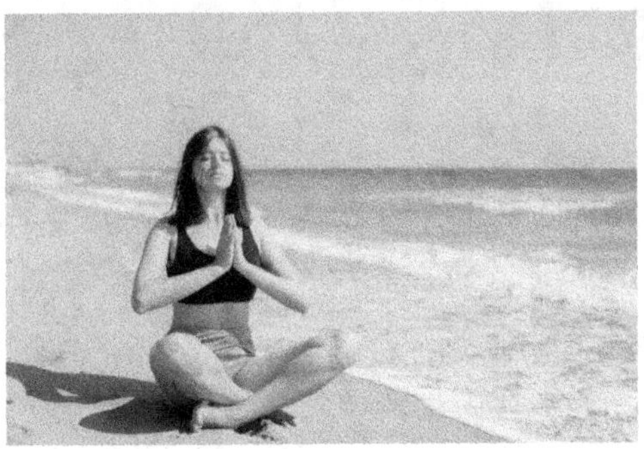

Self Care is the practice of doing different activities to promote your well being. These can be for a short term or a long term period of time. It can be categorized in different subsections: Physical, Mental, Social, Spiritual or Emotional.

It all depends on your needs and what you value the most.

Sample Goal #2
Self Care- continued

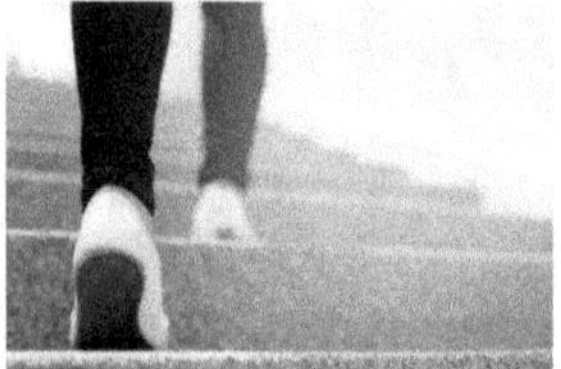

Physical self-care:

- Exercise (walking, swimming, gym)
- get enough sleep
- eat healthy
- if you take medications, make sure you take them and you go to all your medical appointments

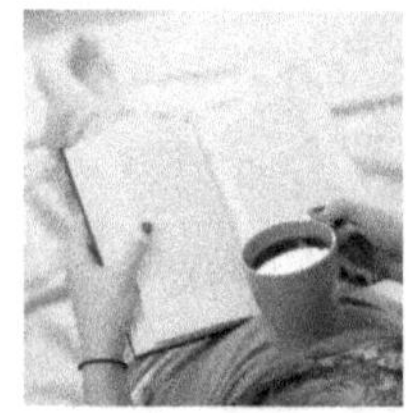

Mental self-care.

- reading a book
- learning something new based on your interest
- doing puzzles
- watching inspiring movies or shows

Sample Goal #2
Self Care- continued

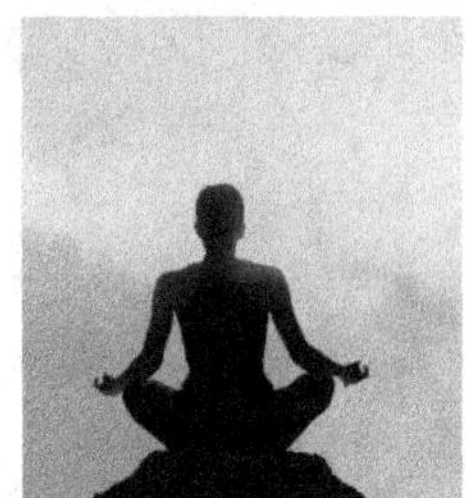

Spiritual Self Care.
- Meditate
- Practice yoga
- If you are religious
    - go to religious services
    - praying
    - going to retreats
- Read spiritual books

Social Self Care.
- Make time to go out with your friends
- spend time with your family
- spend time with your significant other

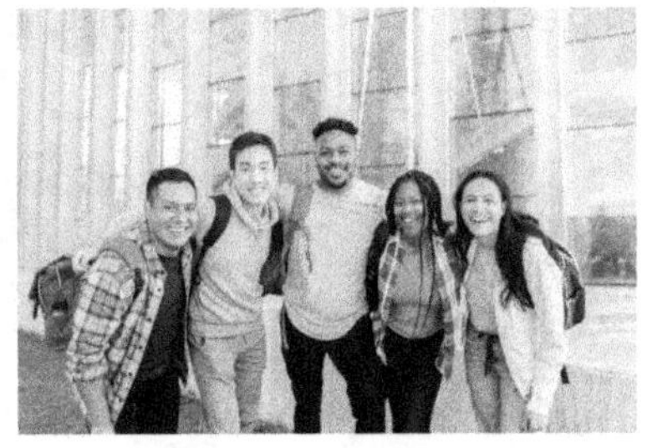

Sample Goal #2
Self Care- continued

Emotional Self Care.

- Have positive affirmations

reading a book or listen to a podcast with positive affirmations

- when you wake up in the morning start with a positive phrase: ex: today will be a good day, today I will accomplish everything I need, I know I can do anything,
- Take care of your appearance
- Go to a spa- try massages, waxing, doing your nails
- try a different hair style, hair color
- go shopping- try different styles
- healthy coping skills for stress, anxiety, or anger
- relaxation exercises such as breathing exercises or meditation
- listening to calming music
- go for a walk
- talk to your trusted support (family or friend)
- self -talk
- have a journal to write what you are feeling
- ask for help

Sample Goal #3
Boost your energy level

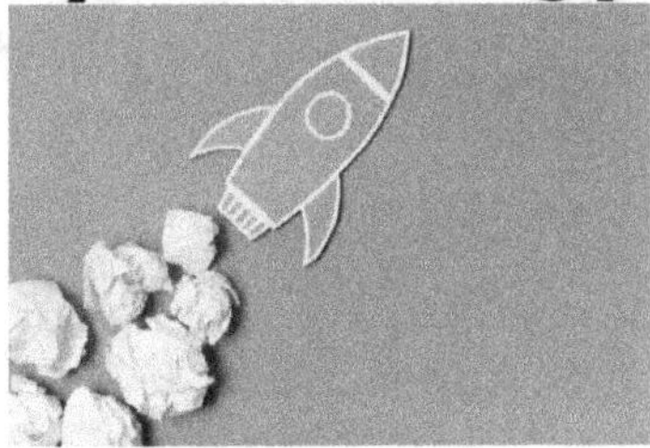

Strategies that can help

1) Get better sleep- Remember that during your sleep your body cells are repairing themselves. Your brain is getting the break it needs to allow you to be able to learn new things and retain more information.

2) Eat healthy- Having a healthy meal goes a long way! Eating well (fruits, vegetables, low sugar, low salt, watching out for fried food) can help you feel more energized to do the things you need.

3) Exercise- You can go to the gym and do several exercises routines. But if you are like me, just take a walk. You can also jog or run or go swimming. Just need to keep your body moving to help your muscles thus boosting your mood.

Sample Goal #3
Boost your energy level continued..

Strategies that can help

4) Listening to your favorite tunes can help you feel good and change your mood.

5) Talking to your family and friends. Talking to someone you trust can help you by expressing your emotions. Keeping feelings inside is not good especially if those feelings are bringing you down. Having a friendly conversation can help you release those thoughts and get good advice.

6) Eat chocolate! Scientists believe that dark chocolate can increase your serotonin (the happy hormone) levels. This hormone helps with better sleep and better mood. But remember that too much of anything is not good. So, do not overdo it.

Chapter 4
Sample Plans

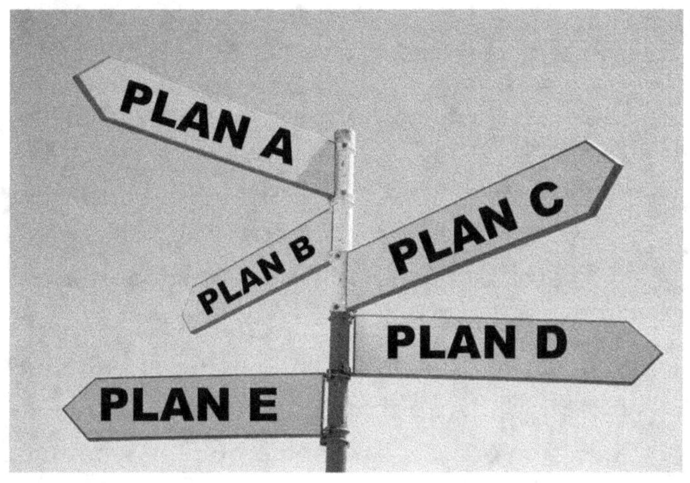

Sample Plan #1
Reducing my stress levels

I will share two plans that I have done and worked for me. Now, they are part of my life routine. If they worked for me, then they may work for you too! I did these two plans around the same time since they went hand in hand.

Remember to adjust the plan to fit your needs.

Step 1: My SMART goal.
My husband and I both work to support our family. We have three young children. Having to wake up at 5am and return home around 5pm while making sure that our kids were taken care of, it is no easy task. Keeping track of what the kids are eating, wearing, their school and their appointments plus our house responsibilities (bills, laundry, supermarket, cleaning) was stressful. I felt we had no time. I felt that 24 hours in a day was not enough to do all the things we needed to do. So, we decided that we needed a plan. We needed a schedule. We needed to be able to manage our time effectively.

Step 2: Reflect to motivate.

I struggle with last minute changes. I know that I feel less stress when I know in advance what I need to do and by when I need to do it. My husband does so much better with spontaneity and last-minute things. That is definitely NOT my case. I need a clear goal, a clear method, and a clear plan to be able to feel successful. I am a very visual and tactile person so, I knew that I needed something that was tangible, visually appealing, and simple to follow.

Step 3: Making my plan.

I started to look for ways to have a visual schedule that could work for me. I have tried planners, and they were not my forte. After looking, I found a magnetic dry erase calendar set that I could place on my fridge. The set brought a monthly calendar, a weekly schedule, and a shopping list. I figured that this may work for me since I can place all my appointments on the calendar, I could write what I needed on the shopping list as soon as it was finished, and in the weekly schedule I could be more specific on what I needed to do that week.
This calendar will always be visible since I am always going to the kitchen. We will always need to get something from the fridge. It was unavoidable. So, I decided to try it. I told myself that I was giving myself a month to see how it worked.

Step 4: Executing my plan.

I started my plan in the month of November
to be revised in December. I bought a dry
erase marker, and I wrote all my
appointments, schools' activities, my
children's school schedule, and even my job
schedule (days I was off due to holidays). I
can say that I saw this calendar all the time!
It was always in my face. I was constantly
reminded of what was coming up.
I also started writing the list of the things I
needed to buy. Also, a tremendous help since
I was writing them in real time.

Step 5: Reflection

This was an incredibly good start. I was constantly reminded of all the activities coming up and there was not surprise. By the end of the month even my husband was looking at the calendar. I also liked the shopping list. My husband and I were both writing things on the list when needed. When I had to go to the supermarket it was less stressful since I knew what we ran out of in the house. And for the first time, I did not forget anything at the supermarket. That was a huge win. I did not use the weekly schedule as I should have. I used it the first week but by the second week I forgot to write things. So, I decided to keep the calendar and the shopping list on my fridge since they did work.

Now a year later, it has become a routine. I always write what I need for the month and even go to my calendar when I am on the phone booking kids' appointments. I know that many people like having the calendar on their phones but for me this physical calendar works so much better. Many will say that they do not want to write on the calendar every month but, the more you write things, the more you remember. I like technology but sometimes going to old school is not bad.

Sample Plan #2
Boosting my energy level

Remember to adjust the plan to fit your needs.

Step 1: My SMART goal.

Like many parents, the struggle of working and raising our children can leave us with no energy at the end of the day. Weekdays are for working, kids going to school, any extra activities the kids have, and any appointments. The weekends are for supermarket, laundry, and cleaning. This is exhausting! By the end of the night, I was done. My energy levels were below zero. Some days even getting to the shower was a struggle. I had no energy. I needed to do something to boost my energy and have some time for myself.

Step 2: Reflect to motivate.

The truth is that I had more energy before the kids. FYI parents, it is okay to admit this! It does not make you bad parents! I was younger, less responsibilities, less worries. Now with a family, the level of responsibility has increased a thousand times fold. I love and adore my husband and my kids, but the reality is that they take away a lot of my energy. I needed to do something to increase my energy levels. This will reduce my stress thus improving my mood as well.

I started researching for ways that could help me. I read many articles on how to boost my energy. Most gave me promising ideas (eat better, sleep more, reduce stress, read a book, go out with friends) but my response was the same: "when will I have time to do this."

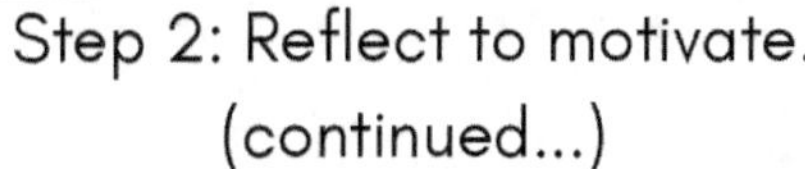

Step 2: Reflect to motivate.
(continued...)

From Monday through Friday, I was a robot-wake up, prepare lunches, get ready, get kids ready, go to school, go to work, get home, prepare dinner, kids' homework, kids' bath, kids' bedtime, our bedtime, and then repeat the next day. So, time was not on my side. My stress was going up and my energy going down.

Then I started reducing my stress (see goal #1) and thus decided to also work on my energy level. Since my plan to reduce stress was monthly and reducing stress was a way to boost energy, I figured that I could work on this as well. After thinking about what can boost energy and increase mood, I realized that I was not eating a well-balanced meal. I sometimes would skip meals and just eat snacks.

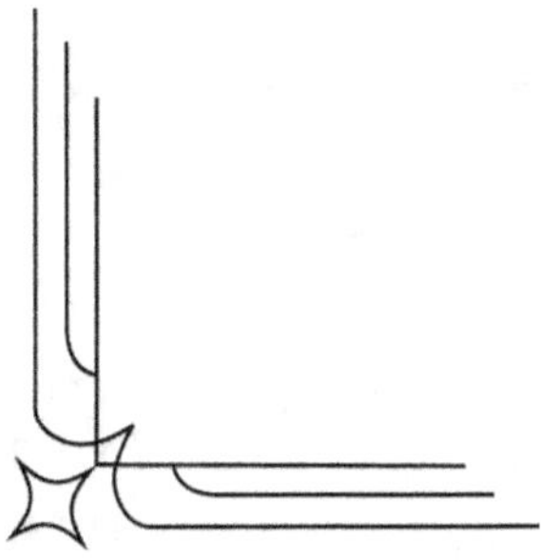
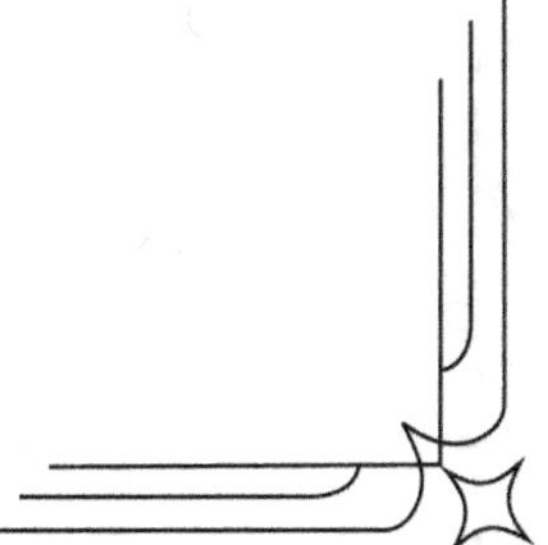

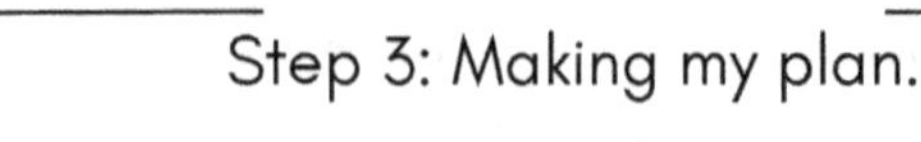

Step 3: Making my plan.

1. I decided to stop snacking on junk food all the time.
2. I made a list of healthy snacks that I could have (especially when I am driving since I have a long ride from work)
3. Instead of buying fast food when I got out of work, I would take lunch from home.
4. In the supermarket, I will buy more fruits and vegetables (also for my kids to eat healthier) and proteins
5. I decided to think in advance about what we will eat for dinner for the week. (not meal prep since I have tried that before and it did not work out for me)
6. I would give myself a month to see if my energy levels have gone up.
7. I would know they went up if I was less tired at the end of the day, I was more energetic in the morning, and my body hurt less.

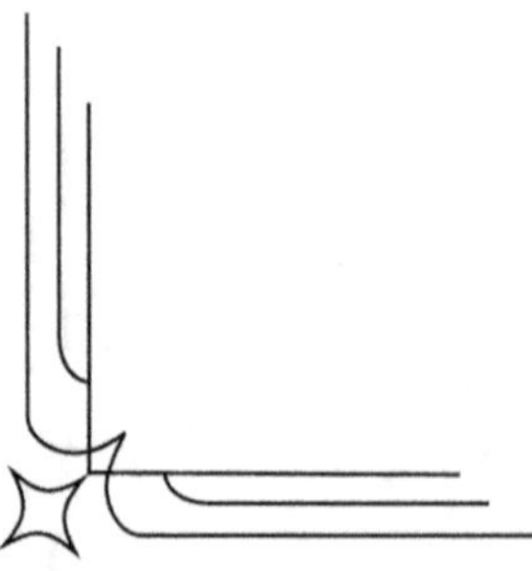
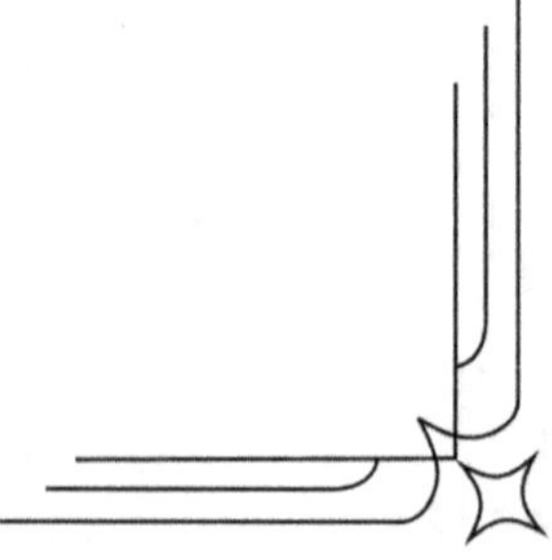

Step 4: Executing my plan.

With my plan set, I started. To help me, I recruited my husband. At the end of the day, he will ask me how my energy was. Then at the end of the week we talked about my mood.

For this plan, if you do not have someone helping you, then you could benefit from having a mini diary. This could be a notepad, stickies, or an app on your phone. Just make sure you have a way to check on how this is going.

I started buying more fruits and vegetables and incorporating them for my snacks and for my children's snacks as well. I started including more vegetables for dinner. Also, drinking more water and less sugary drinks. Knowing what I was going to cook for the week also helped me plan to have healthier options. I was able to write what I needed on my shopping list and thus get them.

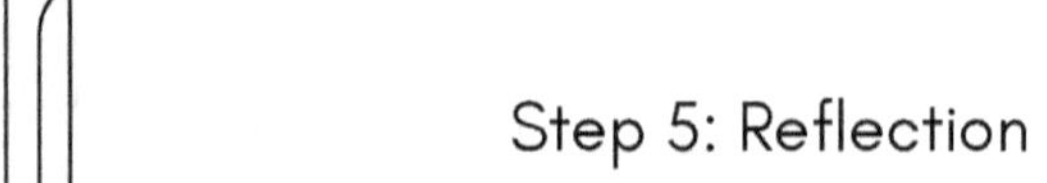

Step 5: Reflection

After a month, I reflected on my goal. My energy level did go up and my mood did change. Having more energy increased the time it took me to accomplish different tasks. I (as well as my family) am eating healthier and drinking more water. I can do more things with my kids and my husband. I have the energy to even watch a movie with my husband after the kids go to sleep.

Eating healthier has become a routine in my house as well. My kids are eating more fruits and vegetables and are a little less fussy with their food. They love sweets like any child but, I can say that they are asking for fruits every day.

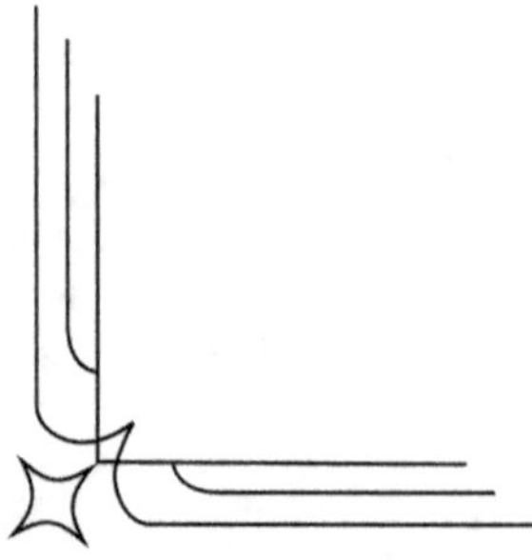

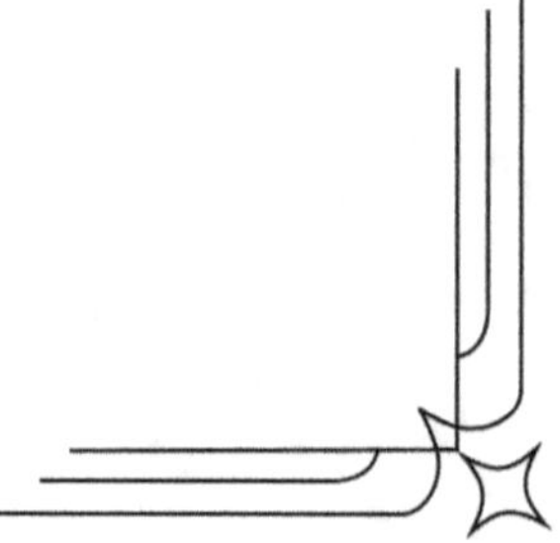

Hope the strategies in this
book were able to help you as
it has helped me..
Thank you for your support!

Ana Soto

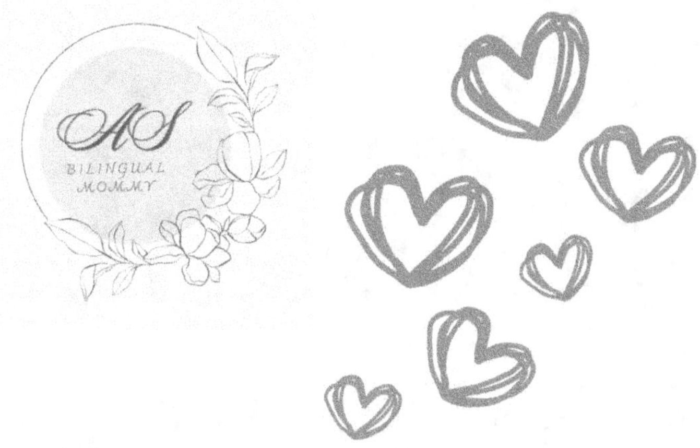